LOW CARB

DIARY

BY

DENISE BLAIR

Counting carbs isn't that hard – most packages, most processed foods are labeled with carb content. Meat is a no-brainer – it does not contain carbs unless you dip in batter or coat with flour or bread crumbs. The things to avoid on a low carb diet are all things containing sugar: pop, ice cream, cookies, cakes, pies, chocolate, packaged treats, donuts, sweetened coffee drinks, muffins, pancakes, syrup, and the list goes on and on. We are an increasing "girth" society due to processed and sugar sweetened manufactured foods. Shopping the outer isles of the grocery store is where you want to be (except bakery).

Alcohol is full of carbs – so if you want to lose weight – avoid it.

Potatoes, pasta and rice contains carbs – so use in moderation.

This is a 30 day low carb/sugar free diary – to get you on the right track and reduce unwanted weight.

My Low Carb Diary

Day 1: _____

Meat 0 0 0 0

Dairy 0 0 0 0

Veggies 0 0 0 0

Carbs – 0 0 0 (bread, pasta, rice)

Fill in the circles as you go through your day. Each circle represents a fist sized or cup sized serving.

Dairy represents eggs, milk, and cheese.

Suggested meals:

Breakfast: eggs and bacon, one slice of buttered toast or half a bagel with cream cheese and half a banana and cup of milk.

Lunch: sandwich such as egg salad, roast beef, ham, turkey, cheese using whole grain bread, ½ apple, and cup of milk.

Dinner choices are numerous and include chicken, beef, fish, or pork, a vegetable and a starch (potatoes, rice, and pasta) plus a salad.

My Low Carb Diary

Day 1: _____

Meat 0 0 0 0

Dairy 0 0 0 0

Veggies 0 0 0 0

Carbs – 0 0 0 (bread, pasta, rice)

Fill in the circles as you go through your day. Each circle represents a fist sized or cup sized serving.

Dairy represents eggs, milk, and cheese.

Suggested meals:

Breakfast: eggs and bacon, one slice of buttered toast or half a bagel with cream cheese and half a banana and cup of milk.

Lunch: sandwich such as egg salad, roast beef, ham, turkey, cheese using whole grain bread, ½ apple, and cup of milk.

Dinner choices are numerous and include chicken, beef, fish, or pork, a vegetable and a starch (potatoes, rice, and pasta) plus a salad.

My Low Carb Diary

Day 1: _____

Meat 0 0 0 0

Dairy 0 0 0 0

Veggies 0 0 0 0

Carbs – 0 0 0 (bread, pasta, rice)

Fill in the circles as you go through your day. Each circle represents a fist sized or cup sized serving.

Dairy represents eggs, milk, and cheese.

Suggested meals:

Breakfast: eggs and bacon, one slice of buttered toast or half a bagel with cream cheese and half a banana and cup of milk.

Lunch: sandwich such as egg salad, roast beef, ham, turkey, cheese using whole grain bread, ½ apple, and cup of milk.

Dinner choices are numerous and include chicken, beef, fish, or pork, a vegetable and a starch (potatoes, rice, and pasta) plus a salad.

My Low Carb Diary

Day 1: _____

Meat 0 0 0 0

Dairy 0 0 0 0

Veggies 0 0 0 0

Carbs – 0 0 0 (bread, pasta, rice)

Fill in the circles as you go through your day. Each circle represents a fist sized or cup sized serving.

Dairy represents eggs, milk, and cheese.

Suggested meals:

Breakfast: eggs and bacon, one slice of buttered toast or half a bagel with cream cheese and half a banana and cup of milk.

Lunch: sandwich such as egg salad, roast beef, ham, turkey, cheese using whole grain bread, ½ apple, and cup of milk.

Dinner choices are numerous and include chicken, beef, fish, or pork, a vegetable and a starch (potatoes, rice, and pasta) plus a salad.

My Low Carb Diary

Day 1: _____

Meat 0 0 0 0

Dairy 0 0 0 0

Veggies 0 0 0 0

Carbs – 0 0 0 (bread, pasta, rice)

Fill in the circles as you go through your day. Each circle represents a fist sized or cup sized serving.

Dairy represents eggs, milk, and cheese.

Suggested meals:

Breakfast: eggs and bacon, one slice of buttered toast or half a bagel with cream cheese and half a banana and cup of milk.

Lunch: sandwich such as egg salad, roast beef, ham, turkey, cheese using whole grain bread, ½ apple, and cup of milk.

Dinner choices are numerous and include chicken, beef, fish, or pork, a vegetable and a starch (potatoes, rice, and pasta) plus a salad.

My Low Carb Diary

Day 1: _____

Meat 0 0 0 0

Dairy 0 0 0 0

Veggies 0 0 0 0

Carbs – 0 0 0 (bread, pasta, rice)

Fill in the circles as you go through your day. Each circle represents a fist sized or cup sized serving.

Dairy represents eggs, milk, and cheese.

Suggested meals:

Breakfast: eggs and bacon, one slice of buttered toast or half a bagel with cream cheese and half a banana and cup of milk.

Lunch: sandwich such as egg salad, roast beef, ham, turkey, cheese using whole grain bread, ½ apple, and cup of milk.

Dinner choices are numerous and include chicken, beef, fish, or pork, a vegetable and a starch (potatoes, rice, and pasta) plus a salad.

My Low Carb Diary

Day 1: _____

Meat 0 0 0 0

Dairy 0 0 0 0

Veggies 0 0 0 0

Carbs – 0 0 0 (bread, pasta, rice)

Fill in the circles as you go through your day. Each circle represents a fist sized or cup sized serving.

Dairy represents eggs, milk, and cheese.

Suggested meals:

Breakfast: eggs and bacon, one slice of buttered toast or half a bagel with cream cheese and half a banana and cup of milk.

Lunch: sandwich such as egg salad, roast beef, ham, turkey, cheese using whole grain bread, ½ apple, and cup of milk.

Dinner choices are numerous and include chicken, beef, fish, or pork, a vegetable and a starch (potatoes, rice, and pasta) plus a salad.

My Low Carb Diary

Day 1: _____

Meat 0 0 0 0

Dairy 0 0 0 0

Veggies 0 0 0 0

Carbs – 0 0 0 (bread, pasta, rice)

Fill in the circles as you go through your day. Each circle represents a fist sized or cup sized serving.

Dairy represents eggs, milk, and cheese.

Suggested meals:

Breakfast: eggs and bacon, one slice of buttered toast or half a bagel with cream cheese and half a banana and cup of milk.

Lunch: sandwich such as egg salad, roast beef, ham, turkey, cheese using whole grain bread, ½ apple, and cup of milk.

Dinner choices are numerous and include chicken, beef, fish, or pork, a vegetable and a starch (potatoes, rice, and pasta) plus a salad.

My Low Carb Diary

Day 1: _____

Meat 0 0 0 0

Dairy 0 0 0 0

Veggies 0 0 0 0

Carbs – 0 0 0 (bread, pasta, rice)

Fill in the circles as you go through your day. Each circle represents a fist sized or cup sized serving.

Dairy represents eggs, milk, and cheese.

Suggested meals:

Breakfast: eggs and bacon, one slice of buttered toast or half a bagel with cream cheese and half a banana and cup of milk.

Lunch: sandwich such as egg salad, roast beef, ham, turkey, cheese using whole grain bread, ½ apple, and cup of milk.

Dinner choices are numerous and include chicken, beef, fish, or pork, a vegetable and a starch (potatoes, rice, and pasta) plus a salad.

My Low Carb Diary

Day 1: _____

Meat 0 0 0 0

Dairy 0 0 0 0

Veggies 0 0 0 0

Carbs – 0 0 0 (bread, pasta, rice)

Fill in the circles as you go through your day. Each circle represents a fist sized or cup sized serving.

Dairy represents eggs, milk, and cheese.

Suggested meals:

Breakfast: eggs and bacon, one slice of buttered toast or half a bagel with cream cheese and half a banana and cup of milk.

Lunch: sandwich such as egg salad, roast beef, ham, turkey, cheese using whole grain bread, ½ apple, and cup of milk.

Dinner choices are numerous and include chicken, beef, fish, or pork, a vegetable and a starch (potatoes, rice, and pasta) plus a salad.

My Low Carb Diary

Day 1: _____

Meat 0 0 0 0

Dairy 0 0 0 0

Veggies 0 0 0 0

Carbs – 0 0 0 (bread, pasta, rice)

Fill in the circles as you go through your day. Each circle represents a fist sized or cup sized serving.

Dairy represents eggs, milk, and cheese.

Suggested meals:

Breakfast: eggs and bacon, one slice of buttered toast or half a bagel with cream cheese and half a banana and cup of milk.

Lunch: sandwich such as egg salad, roast beef, ham, turkey, cheese using whole grain bread, ½ apple, and cup of milk.

Dinner choices are numerous and include chicken, beef, fish, or pork, a vegetable and a starch (potatoes, rice, and pasta) plus a salad.

My Low Carb Diary

Day 1: _____

Meat 0 0 0 0

Dairy 0 0 0 0

Veggies 0 0 0 0

Carbs – 0 0 0 (bread, pasta, rice)

Fill in the circles as you go through your day. Each circle represents a fist sized or cup sized serving.

Dairy represents eggs, milk, and cheese.

Suggested meals:

Breakfast: eggs and bacon, one slice of buttered toast or half a bagel with cream cheese and half a banana and cup of milk.

Lunch: sandwich such as egg salad, roast beef, ham, turkey, cheese using whole grain bread, ½ apple, and cup of milk.

Dinner choices are numerous and include chicken, beef, fish, or pork, a vegetable and a starch (potatoes, rice, and pasta) plus a salad.

My Low Carb Diary

Day 1: _____

Meat 0 0 0 0

Dairy 0 0 0 0

Veggies 0 0 0 0

Carbs – 0 0 0 (bread, pasta, rice)

Fill in the circles as you go through your day. Each circle represents a fist sized or cup sized serving.

Dairy represents eggs, milk, and cheese.

Suggested meals:

Breakfast: eggs and bacon, one slice of buttered toast or half a bagel with cream cheese and half a banana and cup of milk.

Lunch: sandwich such as egg salad, roast beef, ham, turkey, cheese using whole grain bread, ½ apple, and cup of milk.

Dinner choices are numerous and include chicken, beef, fish, or pork, a vegetable and a starch (potatoes, rice, and pasta) plus a salad.

My Low Carb Diary

Day 1: _____

Meat 0 0 0 0

Dairy 0 0 0 0

Veggies 0 0 0 0

Carbs – 0 0 0 (bread, pasta, rice)

Fill in the circles as you go through your day. Each circle represents a fist sized or cup sized serving.

Dairy represents eggs, milk, and cheese.

Suggested meals:

Breakfast: eggs and bacon, one slice of buttered toast or half a bagel with cream cheese and half a banana and cup of milk.

Lunch: sandwich such as egg salad, roast beef, ham, turkey, cheese using whole grain bread, ½ apple, and cup of milk.

Dinner choices are numerous and include chicken, beef, fish, or pork, a vegetable and a starch (potatoes, rice, and pasta) plus a salad.

My Low Carb Diary

Day 1: _____

Meat 0 0 0 0

Dairy 0 0 0 0

Veggies 0 0 0 0

Carbs – 0 0 0 (bread, pasta, rice)

Fill in the circles as you go through your day. Each circle represents a fist sized or cup sized serving.

Dairy represents eggs, milk, and cheese.

Suggested meals:

Breakfast: eggs and bacon, one slice of buttered toast or half a bagel with cream cheese and half a banana and cup of milk.

Lunch: sandwich such as egg salad, roast beef, ham, turkey, cheese using whole grain bread, ½ apple, and cup of milk.

Dinner choices are numerous and include chicken, beef, fish, or pork, a vegetable and a starch (potatoes, rice, and pasta) plus a salad.

My Low Carb Diary

Day 1: _____

Meat 0 0 0 0

Dairy 0 0 0 0

Veggies 0 0 0 0

Carbs – 0 0 0 (bread, pasta, rice)

Fill in the circles as you go through your day. Each circle represents a fist sized or cup sized serving.

Dairy represents eggs, milk, and cheese.

Suggested meals:

Breakfast: eggs and bacon, one slice of buttered toast or half a bagel with cream cheese and half a banana and cup of milk.

Lunch: sandwich such as egg salad, roast beef, ham, turkey, cheese using whole grain bread, ½ apple, and cup of milk.

Dinner choices are numerous and include chicken, beef, fish, or pork, a vegetable and a starch (potatoes, rice, and pasta) plus a salad.

My Low Carb Diary

Day 1: _____

Meat 0 0 0 0

Dairy 0 0 0 0

Veggies 0 0 0 0

Carbs – 0 0 0 (bread, pasta, rice)

Fill in the circles as you go through your day. Each circle represents a fist sized or cup sized serving.

Dairy represents eggs, milk, and cheese.

Suggested meals:

Breakfast: eggs and bacon, one slice of buttered toast or half a bagel with cream cheese and half a banana and cup of milk.

Lunch: sandwich such as egg salad, roast beef, ham, turkey, cheese using whole grain bread, ½ apple, and cup of milk.

Dinner choices are numerous and include chicken, beef, fish, or pork, a vegetable and a starch (potatoes, rice, and pasta) plus a salad.

My Low Carb Diary

Day 1: _____

Meat 0 0 0 0

Dairy 0 0 0 0

Veggies 0 0 0 0

Carbs – 0 0 0 (bread, pasta, rice)

Fill in the circles as you go through your day. Each circle represents a fist sized or cup sized serving.

Dairy represents eggs, milk, and cheese.

Suggested meals:

Breakfast: eggs and bacon, one slice of buttered toast or half a bagel with cream cheese and half a banana and cup of milk.

Lunch: sandwich such as egg salad, roast beef, ham, turkey, cheese using whole grain bread, ½ apple, and cup of milk.

Dinner choices are numerous and include chicken, beef, fish, or pork, a vegetable and a starch (potatoes, rice, and pasta) plus a salad.

My Low Carb Diary

Day 1: _____

Meat 0 0 0 0

Dairy 0 0 0 0

Veggies 0 0 0 0

Carbs – 0 0 0 (bread, pasta, rice)

Fill in the circles as you go through your day. Each circle represents a fist sized or cup sized serving.

Dairy represents eggs, milk, and cheese.

Suggested meals:

Breakfast: eggs and bacon, one slice of buttered toast or half a bagel with cream cheese and half a banana and cup of milk.

Lunch: sandwich such as egg salad, roast beef, ham, turkey, cheese using whole grain bread, ½ apple, and cup of milk.

Dinner choices are numerous and include chicken, beef, fish, or pork, a vegetable and a starch (potatoes, rice, and pasta) plus a salad.

My Low Carb Diary

Day 1: _____

Meat 0 0 0 0

Dairy 0 0 0 0

Veggies 0 0 0 0

Carbs – 0 0 0 (bread, pasta, rice)

Fill in the circles as you go through your day. Each circle represents a fist sized or cup sized serving.

Dairy represents eggs, milk, and cheese.

Suggested meals:

Breakfast: eggs and bacon, one slice of buttered toast or half a bagel with cream cheese and half a banana and cup of milk.

Lunch: sandwich such as egg salad, roast beef, ham, turkey, cheese using whole grain bread, ½ apple, and cup of milk.

Dinner choices are numerous and include chicken, beef, fish, or pork, a vegetable and a starch (potatoes, rice, and pasta) plus a salad.

My Low Carb Diary

Day 1: _____

Meat 0 0 0 0

Dairy 0 0 0 0

Veggies 0 0 0 0

Carbs – 0 0 0 (bread, pasta, rice)

Fill in the circles as you go through your day. Each circle represents a fist sized or cup sized serving.

Dairy represents eggs, milk, and cheese.

Suggested meals:

Breakfast: eggs and bacon, one slice of buttered toast or half a bagel with cream cheese and half a banana and cup of milk.

Lunch: sandwich such as egg salad, roast beef, ham, turkey, cheese using whole grain bread, ½ apple, and cup of milk.

Dinner choices are numerous and include chicken, beef, fish, or pork, a vegetable and a starch (potatoes, rice, and pasta) plus a salad.

My Low Carb Diary

Day 1: _____

Meat 0 0 0 0

Dairy 0 0 0 0

Veggies 0 0 0 0

Carbs – 0 0 0 (bread, pasta, rice)

Fill in the circles as you go through your day. Each circle represents a fist sized or cup sized serving.

Dairy represents eggs, milk, and cheese.

Suggested meals:

Breakfast: eggs and bacon, one slice of buttered toast or half a bagel with cream cheese and half a banana and cup of milk.

Lunch: sandwich such as egg salad, roast beef, ham, turkey, cheese using whole grain bread, ½ apple, and cup of milk.

Dinner choices are numerous and include chicken, beef, fish, or pork, a vegetable and a starch (potatoes, rice, and pasta) plus a salad.

My Low Carb Diary

Day 1: _____

Meat 0 0 0 0

Dairy 0 0 0 0

Veggies 0 0 0 0

Carbs – 0 0 0 (bread, pasta, rice)

Fill in the circles as you go through your day. Each circle represents a fist sized or cup sized serving.

Dairy represents eggs, milk, and cheese.

Suggested meals:

Breakfast: eggs and bacon, one slice of buttered toast or half a bagel with cream cheese and half a banana and cup of milk.

Lunch: sandwich such as egg salad, roast beef, ham, turkey, cheese using whole grain bread, ½ apple, and cup of milk.

Dinner choices are numerous and include chicken, beef, fish, or pork, a vegetable and a starch (potatoes, rice, and pasta) plus a salad.

My Low Carb Diary

Day 1: _____

Meat 0 0 0 0

Dairy 0 0 0 0

Veggies 0 0 0 0

Carbs – 0 0 0 (bread, pasta, rice)

Fill in the circles as you go through your day. Each circle represents a fist sized or cup sized serving.

Dairy represents eggs, milk, and cheese.

Suggested meals:

Breakfast: eggs and bacon, one slice of buttered toast or half a bagel with cream cheese and half a banana and cup of milk.

Lunch: sandwich such as egg salad, roast beef, ham, turkey, cheese using whole grain bread, ½ apple, and cup of milk.

Dinner choices are numerous and include chicken, beef, fish, or pork, a vegetable and a starch (potatoes, rice, and pasta) plus a salad.

My Low Carb Diary

Day 1: _____

Meat 0 0 0 0

Dairy 0 0 0 0

Veggies 0 0 0 0

Carbs – 0 0 0 (bread, pasta, rice)

Fill in the circles as you go through your day. Each circle represents a fist sized or cup sized serving.

Dairy represents eggs, milk, and cheese.

Suggested meals:

Breakfast: eggs and bacon, one slice of buttered toast or half a bagel with cream cheese and half a banana and cup of milk.

Lunch: sandwich such as egg salad, roast beef, ham, turkey, cheese using whole grain bread, ½ apple, and cup of milk.

Dinner choices are numerous and include chicken, beef, fish, or pork, a vegetable and a starch (potatoes, rice, and pasta) plus a salad.

My Low Carb Diary

Day 1: _____

Meat 0 0 0 0

Dairy 0 0 0 0

Veggies 0 0 0 0

Carbs – 0 0 0 (bread, pasta, rice)

Fill in the circles as you go through your day. Each circle represents a fist sized or cup sized serving.

Dairy represents eggs, milk, and cheese.

Suggested meals:

Breakfast: eggs and bacon, one slice of buttered toast or half a bagel with cream cheese and half a banana and cup of milk.

Lunch: sandwich such as egg salad, roast beef, ham, turkey, cheese using whole grain bread, ½ apple, and cup of milk.

Dinner choices are numerous and include chicken, beef, fish, or pork, a vegetable and a starch (potatoes, rice, and pasta) plus a salad.

My Low Carb Diary

Day 1: _____

Meat 0 0 0 0

Dairy 0 0 0 0

Veggies 0 0 0 0

Carbs – 0 0 0 (bread, pasta, rice)

Fill in the circles as you go through your day. Each circle represents a fist sized or cup sized serving.

Dairy represents eggs, milk, and cheese.

Suggested meals:

Breakfast: eggs and bacon, one slice of buttered toast or half a bagel with cream cheese and half a banana and cup of milk.

Lunch: sandwich such as egg salad, roast beef, ham, turkey, cheese using whole grain bread, ½ apple, and cup of milk.

Dinner choices are numerous and include chicken, beef, fish, or pork, a vegetable and a starch (potatoes, rice, and pasta) plus a salad.

My Low Carb Diary

Day 1: _____

Meat 0 0 0 0

Dairy 0 0 0 0

Veggies 0 0 0 0

Carbs – 0 0 0 (bread, pasta, rice)

Fill in the circles as you go through your day. Each circle represents a fist sized or cup sized serving.

Dairy represents eggs, milk, and cheese.

Suggested meals:

Breakfast: eggs and bacon, one slice of buttered toast or half a bagel with cream cheese and half a banana and cup of milk.

Lunch: sandwich such as egg salad, roast beef, ham, turkey, cheese using whole grain bread, ½ apple, and cup of milk.

Dinner choices are numerous and include chicken, beef, fish, or pork, a vegetable and a starch (potatoes, rice, and pasta) plus a salad.

My Low Carb Diary

Day 1: _____

Meat 0 0 0 0

Dairy 0 0 0 0

Veggies 0 0 0 0

Carbs – 0 0 0 (bread, pasta, rice)

Fill in the circles as you go through your day. Each circle represents a fist sized or cup sized serving.

Dairy represents eggs, milk, and cheese.

Suggested meals:

Breakfast: eggs and bacon, one slice of buttered toast or half a bagel with cream cheese and half a banana and cup of milk.

Lunch: sandwich such as egg salad, roast beef, ham, turkey, cheese using whole grain bread, ½ apple, and cup of milk.

Dinner choices are numerous and include chicken, beef, fish, or pork, a vegetable and a starch (potatoes, rice, and pasta) plus a salad.

My Low Carb Diary

Day 1: _____

Meat 0 0 0 0

Dairy 0 0 0 0

Veggies 0 0 0 0

Carbs – 0 0 0 (bread, pasta, rice)

Fill in the circles as you go through your day. Each circle represents a fist sized or cup sized serving.

Dairy represents eggs, milk, and cheese.

Suggested meals:

Breakfast: eggs and bacon, one slice of buttered toast or half a bagel with cream cheese and half a banana and cup of milk.

Lunch: sandwich such as egg salad, roast beef, ham, turkey, cheese using whole grain bread, ½ apple, and cup of milk.

Dinner choices are numerous and include chicken, beef, fish, or pork, a vegetable and a starch (potatoes, rice, and pasta) plus a salad.

My Low Carb Diary

Day 1: _____

Meat 0 0 0 0

Dairy 0 0 0 0

Veggies 0 0 0 0

Carbs – 0 0 0 (bread, pasta, rice)

Fill in the circles as you go through your day. Each circle represents a fist sized or cup sized serving.

Dairy represents eggs, milk, and cheese.

Suggested meals:

Breakfast: eggs and bacon, one slice of buttered toast or half a bagel with cream cheese and half a banana and cup of milk.

Lunch: sandwich such as egg salad, roast beef, ham, turkey, cheese using whole grain bread, ½ apple, and cup of milk.

Dinner choices are numerous and include chicken, beef, fish, or pork, a vegetable and a starch (potatoes, rice, and pasta) plus a salad.

www.ingramcontent.com/pod-product-compliance
Lightning Source LLC
Chambersburg PA
CBHW070243290526
45789CB00004B/1738